Maalej Bayene
Weli Manel

Dilated cardiomyopathies in children

Maalej Bayene
Weli Manel

Dilated cardiomyopathies in children

ScienciaScripts

Imprint

Any brand names and product names mentioned in this book are subject to trademark, brand or patent protection and are trademarks or registered trademarks of their respective holders. The use of brand names, product names, common names, trade names, product descriptions etc. even without a particular marking in this work is in no way to be construed to mean that such names may be regarded as unrestricted in respect of trademark and brand protection legislation and could thus be used by anyone.

Cover image: www.ingimage.com

This book is a translation from the original published under ISBN 978-620-6-72289-2.

Publisher:
Sciencia Scripts
is a trademark of
Dodo Books Indian Ocean Ltd. and OmniScriptum S.R.L publishing group

120 High Road, East Finchley, London, N2 9ED, United Kingdom
Str. Armeneasca 28/1, office 1, Chisinau MD-2012, Republic of Moldova, Europe
Printed at: see last page
ISBN: 978-620-8-11476-3

DILATED CARDIOMYOPATHY IN CHILDREN

INTRODUCTION

Cardiomyopathies are diseases of the myocardium affecting either systolic or diastolic ventricular function, or both (1). They are a major cause of acute heart failure and a major indication for heart transplantation in children (2).The definition and classification of cardiomyopathies were established and validated by the World Health Organisation in 1995. They are defined as diseases of the myocardium associated with ventricular dysfunction and are classified into four categories according to morphological and haemodynamic characteristics: dilated cardiomyopathy (DCM), hypertrophic cardiomyopathy (HCM), arrhythmogenic right ventricular dysplasia (ARVD) and restrictive cardiomyopathy (RCM) (3). Since then, two other classifications have followed, issued by the American Heart Association in 2006 and the European Society of Cardiology in 2008, based on advances in genetic knowledge of cardiomyopathies. According to the American Heart Association, cardiomyopathies are considered primary when the disease affects the myocardium exclusively or mainly, and secondary when myocardial damage is associated with multi-systemic damage. Primary cardiomyopathies are divided into genetic cardiomyopathies (including : CMH, DAVD, non-compaction of the left ventricle and channalopathies), acquired (Myocarditis) and mixed (CMD and CMR) (4). Similarly, the European Society of Cardiology emphasises the importance of family history and genetic investigation, classifying cardiomyopathies as familial (or genetic) and non-familial (non-genetic). However, this classification does not include rhythm disorders and channalopathies

(5).CMDs are the most common cardiomyopathies in children. Pathophysiologically, they are characterised by dilatation of the left ventricle associated with systolic dysfunction leading to then to cardiac congestion (6). Ultrasound diagnostic criteria have been established to clearly define CMD in children: The left ventricle is dilated, generally thin-walled, and contracts poorly. The diameter shortening fraction is very low, generally less than 25%, with a systolic stress index of less than 20%. There is often a functional mitral leak due to dilatation of the annulus (7).A distinction should be made between constitutional forms (true cardiomyopathies), which affect the structures of the myocyte itself and in particular the contractile or cytoskeletal elements, and acquired or secondary forms (cardiopathies) in which an extra-myocardial factor is responsible for the myocardial damage (infectious, toxic, ischaemic, etc.) (6). Because it has a guarded prognosis, CMD in children requires a well-codified diagnostic strategy based on current advances in exploratory methods, essentially Doppler ultrasound, magnetic resonance imaging and molecular biology. All these advances contribute to a better understanding of the disease and improved quality of care.

EPIDEMIOLOGY

CMD is the most common cardiomyopathy in newborns and infants
(6). Despite its guarded prognosis, its demographics remain uncertain
(1).In adults, the annual incidence of CMD has been estimated at 6 to
8/100,000 (6). However, it is certainly underestimated in children,
given the large number of sudden deaths secondary to DCM not
identified by systematic autopsy.

In 2003, the American Childhood Cardiomyopathy Registry published
an annual incidence of cardiomyopathy of 1.13 per 100,000 infants
and children, highlighting differences according to race, sex and
region. It was significantly higher in infants under one year of age
than in children and adolescents aged between 1 and 18 years (8.34 vs.
0.70 per 100,000, p<0.001), in black children than in white children
(1.47 vs. 1.06 cases per 100,000, p=0.02) and in boys than in girls
(1.32 vs. 0.92 per 100,000, P<0.001). CMD accounted for 50% of
these cardiomyopathies (8).

A more recent American study reported that the annual incidence of
CMD in North America was around 0.57 cases/100,000 children aged
under 18. This same study also showed that race, sex and age
influence the frequency of the disease. In fact, this study reported a
higher incidence in boys than in girls (0.66 vs 0.47 cases per 100,000;
p <0.001), in blacks than in whites (0.98 vs 0.46 cases per 100,000; p
<0.001) and in infants (< 1 year) than in children (4.40 vs 0.34 cases
per 100,000; p <0.001) (1). Arola et al (9) reported an incidence of
CMD of 0.34 cases per 100,000 children per year and a prevalence of

2.6 cases per 100,000 children in Finland, with a higher frequency in infants of around 3.8 per 100 000 cases per year. A high incidence in infants has also been reported in Australia, reaching 4.76 cases/year/100,000 children (10).

A Korean study reported a prevalence of CMD of 1.39 cases. /100,000 children aged under 15, with an average age at diagnosis of 1 year and a slight male predominance (11).

It is important to study the history of the patient presenting with CMD. The notion of parental consanguinity has been noted in 8.8% to 14.7% of cases, depending on the study (12, 13). In addition, the search for a family history of cardiac disease is an important element in the aetiological search, as it points towards a familial disease requiring a genetic study. Towbin et al (1) reported on a paediatric series of 1426 children with CMD, 27.3% of whom had a family history of cardiac disease. Cardiomyopathy was present in 12.6%, sudden death in 6%, congenital heart disease in 2.2%, arrhythmia in 1.8% and genetic syndromes in 4.7% of cases. Unfortunately, data from the Arab world are virtually non-existent, being limited to a few case reports. Similarly for Tunisia, the absence of a national cardiomyopathy register means that clinicians do not have reliable and informative epidemiological data.

PATHOPHYSIOLOGY

CMD is a maladaptation of myocardial function secondary either to an inability of the heart to respond to excess work (e.g. CMD secondary to an obstruction) or to myocardial failure itself (e.g. metabolic abnormality or myocarditis) (14).

Under normal conditions, the heart has a number of functions:

- Contractility is the heart's ability to develop pressure to eject blood at high pressure into the arterial system. It is directly linked to the stretching capacity of myocardial fibres.

- relaxation is the property that allows the ventricle to actively and effectively lower its pressure below that of the atria to allow rapid filling of the ventricles.

- Cardiac compliance is the relationship between pressure and volume in diastole. As diastole progresses and the ventricle fills with blood, there is little variation in pressure, but above a certain volume, pressure increases rapidly in the ventricle (7).

These properties are well illustrated on a pressure-volume curve (Figure 1).

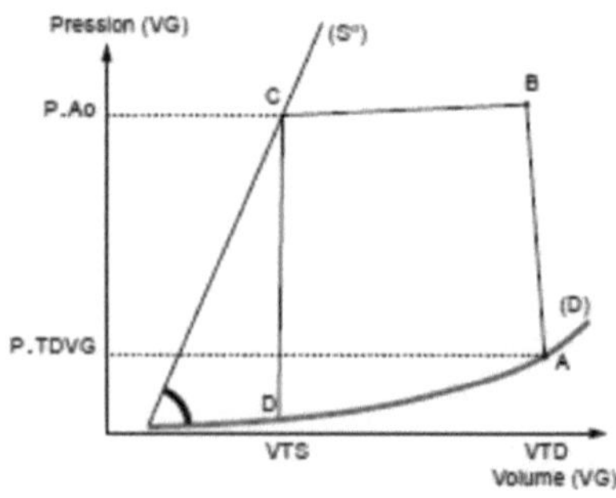

Figure 1: Left ventricular pressure-volume curve.

When the myocardial fibre loses its contractile quality, the myocardial adaptation first takes the form of dilatation to ensure aortic flow and pressure in accordance with Starling's law, which stipulates that the greater the tele-diastolic volume of a ventricle, the greater the energy produced by the ventricle to eject blood. Secondly, compensatory hypertrophy sets in according to Laplace's law. The latter indicates that the parietal stress (CP) or wall stress (the heart's real work) is a direct function of the pressure developed in the cavity (P), the diameter of this cavity (D), i.e. the volume, and inversely a function of the wall thickness E: $CP = P * D/E$ It has been observed that, in order to develop the same pressure, a dilated ventricle must generate greater parietal stress. Myocardial adaptation is therefore based on normalising parietal stress by increasing myocardial mass (7).However, in addition to these myocardial adaptation mechanisms, there are other deleterious processes, in particular myocardial ischaemia resulting from increased oxygen consumption due to myocardial dilation. (7). In addition, impaired myocardial contractility leads to an increase in end-systolic volume and, consequently, end-diastolic volume. The result is an increase in filling pressures and peripheral hypoperfusion. These mechanisms are responsible for cardiac congestion, i.e. heart failure (6). Taken together, these phenomena trigger a neuro-hormonal activation that aims to compensate for these traffic disruptions, but this i s not without risk:

- Activation of the adrenergic system: The increase in adrenergic tone during heart failure has a positive inotropic and chronotropic effect (via cardiacα1 receptors) which can improve cardiac output, but at the cost of an increase in cardiac expenditure. of the myocardium. In addition, the vasoconstriction and increased afterload caused by stimulation of peripheral α1 receptors only aggravates the situation by also increasing the energy expenditure of the heart (6).

- Activation of the renin angiotensin system: Decreased cardiac output and renal hypoperfusion are responsible for activation of the renin angiotensin system. Angiotensin II has a vasoconstrictive effect, enabling normal perfusion pressure to be maintained despite the reduction in cardiac output (15). Similarly, this increase in shift load contributes not only to myocardial hypertrophy but also to vascular wall hypertrophy and increased energy expenditure (16). In addition, this system stimulates sodium reabsorption and thus increases fluid retention, which is not without arrhythmogenic effects (6).

- Arginine-vasopressin is another powerful vasoconstrictor whose levels are increased in heart failure (6).

On the other hand, the production of natriuretic peptides is the most suitable means of combating these deleterious effects. Cardiac natriuretic hormones, including atrial natriuretic peptide (ANP) and brain natriuretic peptide (BNP), as well as their related pro-peptides (proANP and proBNP) represent a group of peptide hormones produced by the heart following the increase in atrial distension pressure to counteract the vasoconstrictive effects and fluid retention of the three systems previously described and also reduce tachycardia (17). It has been shown that a normal level of NT-proBNP has a high negative predictive value for heart failure and that its level is significantly correlated with the severity of heart failure secondary to DCM in children under three years of age (18, 19).

STUDY CLINICAL

The symptoms of DCM are primarily those of heart failure and depend on the extent and abruptness of its onset. Daubeney et al (12) reported that congestive heart failure was the initial clinical presentation in almost 90% of patients, half of whom were admitted to an intensive care unit, and that sudden death was the first manifestation of DCM in almost 5% of cases. Similarly, heart failure was inaugural in 89.7% and 71% of cases respectively in the study by Harmon et al (20) and Towbin et al (1).

1. **Functional signs :**

1.1 Respiratory signs :

Functional respiratory signs are constant and dominate the clinical picture. They range from simple superficial tachypnoea, especially during the effort of feeding, to real respiratory distress with flapping of the wings of the nose and involvement of the intercostal muscles. This is most often seen when heart failure is severe, or when a pulmonary infection is the trigger for decompensation (6).

1.2 General signs

- Fever :

It is generally absent during the state phase. It may be part of a viral myocarditis picture.

- Digestive signs:

Feeding difficulties are often reported. These are directly linked to the intensity of respiratory discomfort and thus have an impact on the child's growth (6, 11).

- **Behavioural problems** such as hypo-responsiveness, apathy or, more rarely, agitation are often present, making the picture more sombre.

2. **Clinical examination**

2.1 Cardiac auscultation :

The tachycardia contrasts with the normal or subnormal temperature. It can point to a cardiac origin if associated with radiological hepatomegaly or cardiomegaly.

Abnormal cardiac auscultation revealing a galloping sound has been reported in several series in the literature with variable frequency. (21,22). It has been suggested that the existence of normal auscultation in the initial phase is a poor prognostic factor (23).

2.6 Hepatomegaly

It is constant in heart failure. It is often very significant and painful (6).

2.7 Oedema and ascites

As with all infant heart failure, oedema and ascites are rare (6).

2.8.2 Blood pressure

Blood pressure is slightly lower but may sometimes be associated with signs of peripheral collapse: pale complexion and/or weak pulse (6).

PARACLINICAL STUDY

Radiological signs :

Cardiomegaly is generally observed and can be assessed by the cardiothoracic ratio. This cardiomegaly mainly affects the ventricles in dilated cardiomyopathy. It is often associated with pulmonary venous stasis or even acute pulmonary oedema (6). (Figure 2)

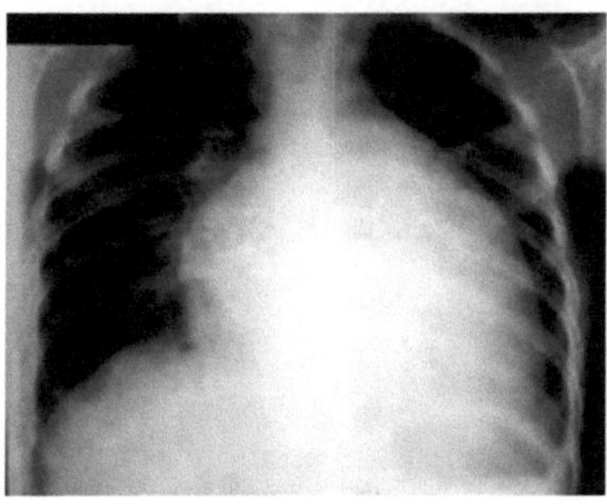

Figure2: Cardiomegaly in a child with CMD

Electrocardiographic signs :

CMD is often associated with conduction and excitability disorders. The P wave axis, atrioventricular and intraventricular conduction and extrasystoles should therefore be checked. We should also look for signs of atrial or ventricular hypertrophy and repolarisation disorders, and even signs of ischaemia (7). In a Chinese study, sinus tachycardia and extrasystoles were the most frequently observed rhythm disorders. Ventricular shortening and ejection fractions were significantly lower in these patients (24).

Ultrasound signs :

Cardiac echocardiography is the key test for the positive and aetiological diagnosis of DCM (7). It is used to assess the systolic and diastolic function of the heart. I n addition to studying cardiac architecture, Doppler allows non-invasive haemodynamic studies to estimate pulmonary pressures and cardiac output. During CMD, the left ventricle is dilated, generally with a thin wall, and contracts poorly. The diameter shortening fraction is very low, generally less than 25% compared with a normal value of 33 ± 3%. The wall is thin, generally less than 5 mm thick in diastole, with a systolic stress index (wall thickness/chamber diameter in telesystole) of less than 20% compared with a normal of 40%. There is often a functional mitral leak secondary to dilatation of the annulus (7). "The American Society of Echocardiography Pediatric and Congenital Heart Disease Council recommends two geometric methods for assessing left ventricular size and function: a linear approach and a volumetric approach. The linear method involves measuring diameters and wall thickness using two-dimensional imaging in TM (or 2D) mode and calculating the shortening fraction. The volumetric method, on the other hand, involves measuring volumes from a 4-cavity apical section using Simpson's method (25). (Figure 3).

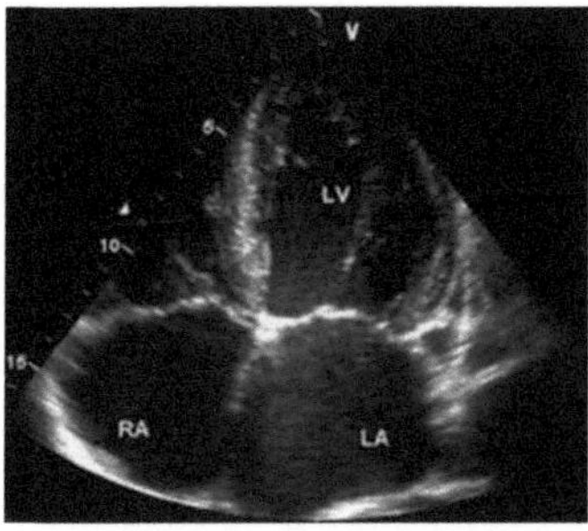

Figure 3: Dilated cardiomyopathy on 2D echocardiography: dilation
of the LV.

Tierney et al (26) showed that for children with DCM, volumetric measurements had better reproducibility compared with two-dimensional and surface methods, when the assessment was not carried out by the same personnel. In addition, some authors have shown that right ventricular systolic and diastolic functions are also affected by left ventricular dysfunction, which warrants ultrasound evaluation (27, 28).

Cardiac MRI :

MRI is a highly effective tool for studying the anatomy and function of the heart. It is currently the reference technique for quantifying left and right ventricular volumes thanks to precise geometric measurements with excellent reproducibility (29). The images that can be observed are local or total hyper-signal in T2-weighted sequences, and after injection of gadolinium, early or late enhancement in T1 sequences (30). Compared with ultrasound, MRI has the advantage of being able to detect the presence of any fibrosis in the heart thanks to this late enhancement (29).Raimondi et al (31) have reported that MRI can predict the course of DCM, as they have shown that the presence of signs of myocardial inflammation on MRI and the elevation of troponin at the time of diagnosis of DCM in affected children are both predictive of LV recovery. Finally, MRI is useful for diagnosing intracardiac thrombi, which remain in hyposignal and do not enhance even in the late stages (32). Figure 4

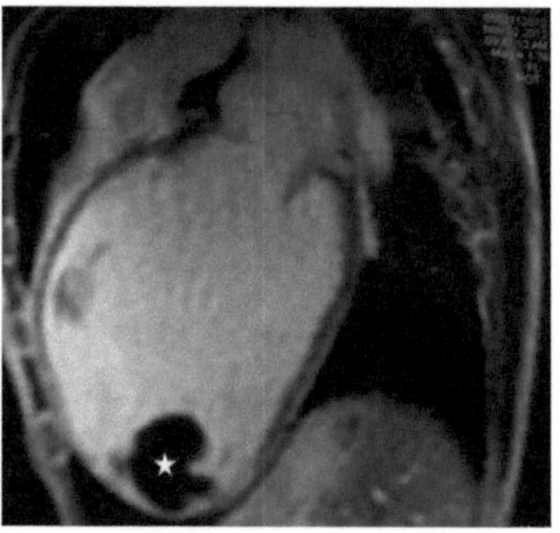

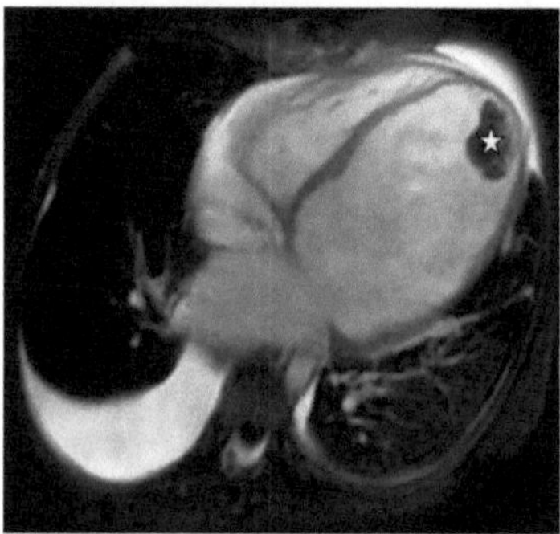

Figure 4: Cardiac MRI after injection of Gadolinium: longitudinal section on the left and transverse section on the right showing two left intra-ventricular thrombi (*), one apical (22x16mm) and one adhering to the anterior wall of the left ventricle (25x6mm).

Cardiac catheterisation :

As an invasive examination, cardiac catheterisation is performed less and less frequently (7).

Cardiac biopsy :

Endomyocardial biopsy (EMB) is a diagnostic tool for assessing myocardial damage and detecting graft rejection after heart transplantation (33, 34).

Although it has been performed quite frequently in adults for some years now, paediatric experience is still not widespread, especially in small infants (35,36).

Its main aim is to differentiate between active viral myocarditis defined as histological evidence of myocardial inflammation associated with a positive PCR on the myocardial sample and acute idiopathic myocarditis defined by the presence of myocardial inflammatory infiltrates associated with myocyte degeneration and non-ischaemic necrosis with a negative PCR (35).

According to Gesuete et al (37), myocardial biopsy is useful in the case of viral myocarditis as it allows PCR of the viral genome to be performed on the sample, thus confirming the diagnosis and guiding treatment.

On the other hand, Brighenti et al (38) reported that BEM enabled an aetiological diagnosis in 63% of cases, and contributed to a therapeutic adaptation in 29.2% of cases. Nishikawa et al (39) showed that the myocardial index, assessed as a function of the presence of fibrosis, variation in myocyte size, muscle bundle disarrangement and mononuclear cell infiltration, was significantly higher in children than in adults. BEM is not without risk, as the patient is exposed to cardiac perforation, thrombosis, haemorrhage or rhythm and conduction disorders, especially when performed on small infants. This risk varies from 12 to 15% depending on the series, reaching 27% in infants under 6 months of age (38, 40).

AETIOLOGIES

CMDs in children represent a heterogeneous group of diseases with multiple aetiologies united by a common clinical presentation of a dilated, poorly contractile heart, generally accompanied by heart failure (41).

The aetiological approach is based first and foremost on a well-directed interview, followed by a thorough clinical examination, with particular emphasis on the search for extra-cardiac damage, and finally on the use of high-performance complementary tests.

In the case of any CMD in a child, the first thing to do is to rule out secondary causes, the diagnosis of which is often obvious when the child has taken a toxic drug (anthracycline), or is already being monitored for a valvular anomaly, coarctation of the aorta or a rhythm disorder, or when there are signs of myocardial ischaemia on the electrocardiogram. (7) It is also important to look for an infectious or inflammatory syndrome, pointing to viral or immunological disease.

However, the etiological search for a primary CMD is much more difficult, but can be guided in this context by the following anamnestic and clinical elements:

- The search for similar cases or deaths at an early age in the family. The family investigation is an important step not only in the aetiological approach, but also in the specific screening of other family members and the proposal of genetic counselling for the parents concerning the risk of recurrence, which is only possible when the aetiology of the cardiomyopathy is well known (12).

- The search for skeletal muscle damage points to myopathies, mitochondrial abnormalities or carnitine deficiency.

- The search for extracardiac involvement other than muscular involvement suggests mitochondrial cytopathy or another generalised metabolic disorder (42-43).

A- Secondary dilated cardiomyopathies :

1. Dilated cardiomyopathy secondary to systolic or diastolic overload of the heart:

It is most common in neonates and young infants. Systolic overload is secondary to a left-sided obstruction represented by coarctation of the aorta, aortic stenosis or arterial hypertension (14). Cardiac auscultation, pulse palpation and blood pressure measurement are therefore of great importance in guiding the diagnosis (7).

On the other hand, long-standing left-right shunts, mitral or aortic leaks and arteriovenous fistulas may be responsible for diastolic volume overload, ultimately leading to DCM (14).

2. Dilated cardiomyopathy secondary to a coronary anomaly :

The most common form is birth defect of the left coronary artery. It generally affects infants between 2 and 5 months of age. Diagnosis is based on the ECG, which should be performed systematically in the presence of any CMD and which shows signs of necrosis or ischaemia (Q wave in D1-VL, sub-endocardial ischaemia from V1 to V4). Doppler ultrasonography confirms the anomaly at the origin of the coronary artery, showing a dilated right coronary artery and, above all, a continuous flow in the pulmonary artery where the left coronary artery joins (7). Other rarer anomalies may be responsible for myocardial ischaemia progressing to DCM: Atresia of the left ostium,

Kawasaki disease with thrombosed aneurysms stenosis or complete obstruction of a coronary artery after reimplantation during large vessel transposition surgery, neonatal ischaemia following perinatal asphyxia and sickle cell anaemia (14).

3. Dilated cardiomyopathy secondary to rhythm or conduction disorders:

These are most often atrial rhythm disorders, such as tachysystole or atrial flutter, which can manifest in utero as foeto-placental hydrops, or show up after birth as hypokinetic CMD if the rhythm disorder is not detected and treated in time (6).

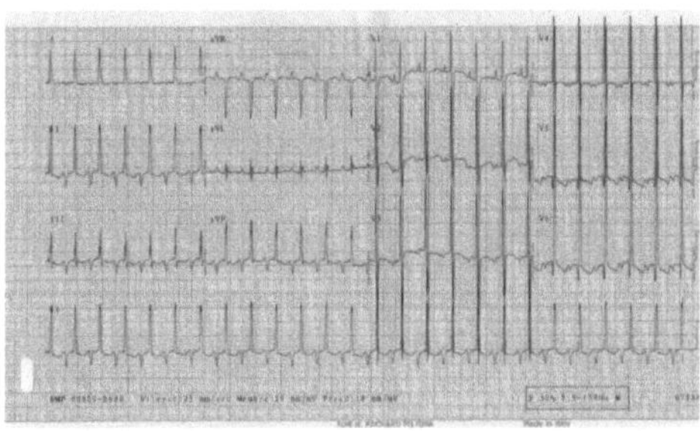

Figure 5: ECG junctional tachycardia in an infant with CMD.

4. Dilated cardiomyopathy secondary to a toxic agent :

The diagnosis is made in the context of anthracycline chemotherapy or radiotherapy. CMD may appear years after the intoxication has stopped (7, 14).

5. Myocarditis

In the aetiological diagnosis of CMD in children, the diagnosis of myocarditis should be made first, because of its frequency, after eliminating secondary CMD and checking for the absence of family history (7,11,12).

It mainly affects infants and children, and may be of infectious or inflammatory origin. Infectious myocarditis is mainly viral (Enterovirus, ParvoB19, HHV6, Adenovirus, CMV, EBV, HSV, influenza virus) but also bacterial (Diphtheria, Tuberculosis, Typhoid, Streptococcus A, Chlamydia, Rickettsioses) or parasitic (Toxoplasmosis, hydatid cyst) (7,44). Inflammatory myocarditis, on the other hand, is rarer in children, and is mainly observed in cases of rheumatic fever, systemic lupus erythematosus or, even more rarely, in cases of sarcoidosis, Churg Strauss syndrome or coeliac disease (44,45). The spectrum of clinical presentation is very broad, ranging from a simple increase in cardiac enzymes to cardiogenic shock with severe rhythm disorders (7).

The difficulty lies in differentiating between viral and inflammatory myocarditis, given the resulting differences in treatment. Proof of viral infection is difficult to obtain, even with the use of a non-harmless endomyocardial biopsy and the viral genome amplification (PCR) technique (7). Viral serology is of little value because of the frequency of viral infections in children, and it is therefore necessary to confirm seroconversion by taking two samples 15 days apart (46).

Daubeney et al (12) have shown that the results of viral identification by PCR on tracheal samples correlate well with those obtained from myocardial or lower respiratory tract samples. The mainstay of treatment is the management of acute heart failure. The value of corticosteroid therapy and venoglobulin infusions has been studied by some teams, with controversial results (44,47). Similarly, there are no studies showing a clear benefit from antiviral infusions (44). Finally, the prognosis for myocarditis is better than for other causes of DCM, but remains unpredictable and only a third of cases progress to recovery with ad integrum restitution (7).

B- Primary cardiomyopathies :

1. Metabolic diseases :

Metabolic investigation is an essential part of the aetiological search for CMD in children, particularly to look for L-carnitine deficiency, which is a metabolic disease that can be cured by providing L-carnitine (7). In the myocardium, carnitine is essential for the beta oxidation of fatty acids, a source of energy for cardiomyocytes (48). Plasma free carnitine levels of less than 20 µmol/L or total carnitine levels of less than 30 µmol/L indicate a carnitine deficiency (6). Other metabolic diseases that may be responsible for DCM are other fatty acid oxidation abnormalities and mitochondrial cytopathies (respiratory chain deficiencies). The prevalence of metabolic abnormalities in CMD varies from 4 to 11% depending on the study (1,2,12). Towbin et al (1) reported that among patients with CMD of metabolic origin, 46% had mitochondrial cytopathy, 24% had Barth's syndrome and 11% had primary carnitine deficiency. The search for a metabolic anomaly is not always easy, and some so-called idiopathic CMDs in fact conceal an inborn error of metabolism (49).

2. Familial or genetic forms

Familial forms of CMD are characterised by great heterogeneity, both genotypic and phenotypic. Their frequency has increased in recent years with advances in molecular biology, affecting up to 20-35% of CMDs (2, 50). It is therefore essential to carry out a family investigation, including a family tree, in the event of any CMD in a child with an affected relative (7). In addition, Nugent et al (10) have shown that children with familial CMD are significantly younger than those with non-familial CMD. Inheritance may be autosomal dominant, autosomal recessive, X-linked or mitochondrial, i.e. exclusively maternal (2). The autosomal dominant form is the most common. The first two genes involved in familial CMD are the gene coding for cardiac actin and the gene coding for dystrophin (51). The gene coding for cardiac actin is the first gene involved in autosomal dominant forms of the disease (52). Depending on the chromosomal location of this gene and the type of mutation, CMD may be isolated or associated with rhythm or conduction disorders or mitral valve prolapse (52,53).

In contrast, the X-linked form of CMD is due to deletions, duplications or point mutations localised in the dystrophin gene (51). These dystrophinopathies are mainly represented by Duchenne and Becker myopathies, Emery-Dreifus myopathies, limb-girdle muscular dystrophies, Barth's syndrome and Friedreich's ataxia (51). The diagnosis of CMD secondary to neuromuscular diseases was made in 26% of cases in the study by Towbin et al (1).

Since then, several genes have been implicated in childhood CMD. These are genes encoding structural proteins (tafazzin, dsarcoglycans), intermediate filament proteins (desmin) (54), nuclear membrane proteins (emerin, A/C lamins) and sarcomeric proteins (MYBPC3, MYH7, TNNT2, TNNI3, TPM1) (55-56).

Very recently, Zhang et al (57) have shown that polymorphism of the LGAL 3 gene encoding a protein Galectin-3, which plays an important role in modulating cardiac inflammation and fibrosis, may be associated with susceptibility to CMD in a Chinese population.

Management of CMD in children includes treatment of heart failure, specific therapies for each aetiology and heart transplantation in the final stage of the disease.

Treatment of heart failure :

The main aims of treatment for heart failure are to reduce pulmonary congestion by prescribing diuretics, to increase myocardial contractility by inotropes and to reduce afterload by vasodilators.

- General measures :

Nutritional management is extremely important in children with heart failure. Calorie intake should be 150 kcal/kg/day, with protein intake of 1.2 to 1.5 g/kg/day (58). Basic fluid intake should be sufficient but should not exceed 75 to 100 ml/kg/day, while salt intake should be reduced to less than 2 mEq/kg/day and potassium intake should be adjusted according to the results of the blood ionogram, especially if diuretic treatment is prescribed (6).

- Diuretics:

They are the first line of treatment for heart failure in children. Loop diuretics are the most commonly used (59). Furosemide can be prescribed discontinuously at a dose of 1-2mg/Kg / 6-12 hours, but it is more advisable to prescribe it continuously at a dose of 0.1 to 0.4mg/Kg/hour (58).

In the event of prolonged prescription, and especially in the event of failure to respond to loop diuretics, a thiazide diuretic is useful as it acts on the distal part of the renal tubule (59). The prescription of a diuretic may be complicated by hydroelectrolytic disorders (hyponatremia, hypokalemia, hypochloremia and metabolic alkalosis), which should be investigated and corrected as soon as possible. time (58,59). The combination of antialdosterone (spironolactone at a dose of 1-2mg/Kg/day) helps to combat secondary hyperaldosteronism and to spare potassium (59, 6).

- Vasodilators: Converting enzyme inhibitors (CEIs): ACE inhibitors have a mixed vasodilatory effect by reducing afterload and preload. They also combat the development of both myocardial and vascular hypertrophy (6). All these effects have contributed to ACE inhibitors becoming a cornerstone in the treatment of childhood heart failure, reducing symptoms and improving survival (60).

Captopril is the most widely studied ACE inhibitor in children. It can be used in neonates (0.4-1.6 mg / kg / day in 3 divided doses) and infants (0.5-4 mg / kg / day in three divided doses). Enalapril can be proposed for children over 2 years of age (0.1-0.5 mg/kg/day in two doses) (59). The adverse effects of ACE inhibitors may include hypotension, reversible impairment of renal function, oedema, cough and hyperkalaemia.

(59). Furthermore, according to the latest recommendations from the International Society of Heart and Lung Transplantation, angiotensin receptor blockers are reserved for children who do not tolerate ACE inhibitors well (60).

- Beta-blockers:

Beta-blockers were previously completely contraindicated in heart failure, but are now widely prescribed in adults, as they have been shown to improve ejection fraction, slow disease progression and reduce the incidence of sudden death (6). They act by counteracting the deleterious effects of chronic stimulation of the sympathetic system (6, 58). Recent studies have supported the beneficial effect of β-blockers in symptomatic children with LV systolic dysfunction. Treatment should be initiated at a low dose in a hemodynamically stable infant already being treated with diuretic and ACE inhibitor at fixed doses, then the dose is gradually increased (6,60, 61,62).

Carvedilol is the most widely studied beta-blocker. Its initial dose is 0.05 mg / kg / dose (twice daily) and is increased to 0.4-0.5 mg / kg / dose (twice daily) by doubling the dose every fortnight under strict monitoring of blood pressure, heart rate and haemodynamic tolerance. Metoprolol (0.1-0.2 mg / kg / dose twice daily and increased to 1 mg / kg / dose twice daily) or Bisoprolol can be used as an alternative to Carvedilol (58).

- Inotropes :

The inotropes most commonly used in acute heart failure i n children are dopamine, dobutamine and Milrinone, despite the absence of randomised controlled trials confirming their benefit on survival in children. (59). Thus, their prescription is limited to the acute phase, especially in cases of myocarditis, and they are not indicated in the management of chronic heart failure, even while waiting for a transplant (60). Dopamine and dobutamine can be prescribed at a dose of 5-20 microg/Kg/minute (59). Epinephrine and norepinephrine can be prescribed but at the cost of an increase in myocardial oxygen consumption and the risk of rhythm disorders (58).

Milrinone, a phosphodiesterase inhibitor, is an inotrope and a peripheral vasodilator. Hoffman et al (63) have demonstrated its beneficial effect in maintaining cardiac output in children undergoing surgery for congenital heart disease. The loading dose is 25-50 microg/Kg/minute, followed by a maintenance dose of 0.25-1 microg/Kg/minute. Levosimendan is another peripheral inotrope and vasodilator currently being studied, the effects of which some authors believe to be promising (64,65). Digoxin continues to be recommended by the International Society of Heart and Lung Transplantation to relieve symptoms in children with heart and lung transplants. heart failure (60). It is contraindicated in premature babies, renal failure and acute myocarditis. It is generally prescribed orally without a loading dose (8-10 microg/Kg/day). A reduction in dose is required when combined with Carvedilol or Amiodarone, targeting a serum level of 0.5-0.9 ng/ml (66). Furthermore, hydro-electrolytic disorders such as hypokalaemia and hypomagnesaemia should be investigated and rapidly corrected to avoid potentiation of its toxicity and the development of rhythm disorders (59).

- **Anticoagulants :**

Anticoagulation with heparin or warfarin is recommended in patients with CMD complicated by an intra-cavity thrombus, or in cases of a history of thromboembolism or complete arrhythmia due to atrial fibrillation with an ejection fraction of less than 25% (60). Anticoagulation was prescribed in 19% of cases in the study by Towbin et al (1), and in 13.7 % of the study by Daubeney et al (12).

- **Extracardiac assistance :**

Extra cardiac membrane oxygenation (ECMO) is widely used in cases of cardiorespiratory arrest. It can also be used in the event of failure of medical treatment, while awaiting a heart transplant or recovery in the event of an aetiology that is likely to be curable (58,59). It improves survival but can also lead to certain serious complications such as infection, haemorrhage and thrombosis (67).

However, retrospective studies have shown that survival after ECMO indicated for severe myocarditis or other cardiomyopathy, whether awaiting cure or transplantation, did not exceed 65%, with increased mortality in infants or when the duration of use exceeded 14 days. (68, 69, 70,71).

In addition, Almond et al (70) reported that 17% of children who underwent ECMO developed neurological complications. On the other hand, implantation of a left ventricular assist device (VAD) is more indicated for infants and in the event of a longer waiting period. Unfortunately, this technique is not without risk, with a high mortality rate (72,73). Complications such as infection, mediastinal haemorrhage and stroke have been reported (74,75). Schranz et al (76) have reported a new indication for an old method, which is the banding of the pulmonary artery in patients with CMD with preserved right ventricular function, allowing correction of the position of the interventricular septum, with early improvement in contractility and progressive recovery of the ejection fraction. This is a promising technique that can replace mechanical assistance. Post-operative management is straightforward, but further studies are needed to assess long-term results, identify adverse effects associated with pressure overload of the right ventricle, and specify the ideal time for any decerclage (67).

- Therapeutic perspective :

Sian Pincott et al (77) showed in a randomised controlled trial that injection of stem cells into the coronary arteries was a safe and effective technique in children with DCM. Left ventricular volume was significantly reduced 6 months after stem cell injection compared with placebo, reflecting myocardial remodelling.

Specific therapies :

Specific treatments for each aetiology mainly concern secondary CMDs, essentially the management of a rhythm or conduction disorder, surgical treatment of obstructive heart disease or with a major shunt, not forgetting L-carnitine deficiency, which is virtually the only primary CMD to benefit from replacement therapy (59). Moriguchi et al (78) reported the efficacy of plasma exchange in cases of CMD of autoimmune origin.

Heart transplantation :

It is indicated in the final stage of heart failure. However, it is often hampered by the scarcity of donors and referral centres. It certainly improves patient survival, but like all transplants, it can be fraught with complications such as viral infections, acute rejection, arterial hypertension, renal failure, allograft vasculitis and lymphoproliferative syndromes (58,59).

THE PROGNOSIS

The course of CMD and prognostic factors vary considerably from one study to another. It is therefore difficult to establish a precise prognosis. The 5-year survival rate varies between 20 and 84% depending on the study (79,80).The age of the child at diagnosis has been studied as a risk factor in several studies. Daubeney (12) and Gesuete (37) reported in their studies that patients aged over 5 years had an unfavourable outcome with a high risk of death or recourse to heart transplantation. Similarly, Towbin et al (1) have shown that DCM is significantly more frequent in the first year of life, but has a poor prognosis in older children.The initial clinical presentation also influences prognosis. Severe heart failure with a low shortening index requiring the use of inotropes is a poor prognostic factor. (2,12, 37) Another important prognostic factor is the aetiology of DCM. Familial DCM often has a poor prognosis, whereas viral myocarditis has a more favourable prognosis (12, 37, 81).

CONCLUSION

CMD is the most common cardiomyopathy in children. Its incidence is difficult to estimate and national registries need to be set up. In all cases of CMD in children, secondary CMD should first be ruled out, followed by metabolic and genetic research, which is often difficult and demanding. Despite advances in diagnosis and management, the prognosis for childhood CMD remains poor. At the end of this review of the child's CMDs, and in the absence of any element of orientation, a decision-making algorithm is proposed for the aetiological investigation (Figure 6).

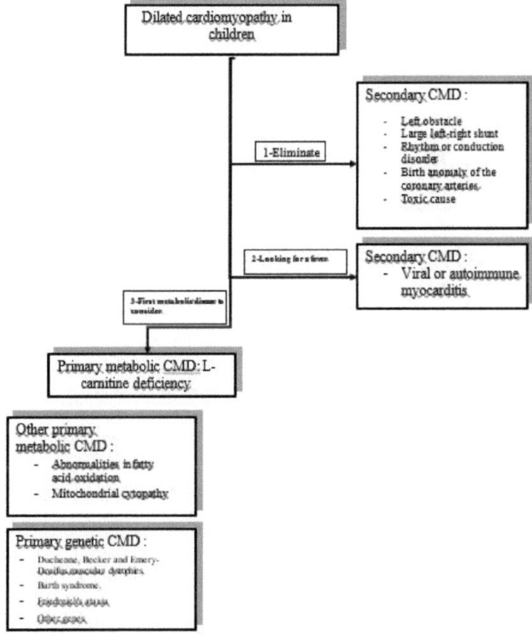

Figure 6: Decision-making algorithm for the aetiological diagnosis of CMD in children

BIBLIOGRAPHY

1. Towbin JA, Lowe AM, Colan SD, Sleeper LA, Orav EJ, Clunie S et al: Incidence, Causes, and Outcomes of Dilated Cardiomyopathy in Children. JAMA. 2006; 296 (15):1867-1876.

2. Williams GD, Hammer GB. Cardiomyopathy in childhood. Curr Opin Anesthesiol. 2011; 24:289-300.

3. Richardson P, McKenna W, Bristow M, Maisch B, Mautner B, O'Connell J, et al. Report of the 1995 World Health Organization / International Society and Federation of Cardiology task force on the definition and classification of cardiomyopathies. Circulation 1996;93:841- 842.

4. Maron BJ, Towbin JA, Thiene G, Antzelevitch C, Corrado D, Arnett D, et al. American Heart Association; Council on Clinical Cardiology, Heart Failure and Transplantation Committee; Quality of Care and Outcomes Research and Functional Genomics and Translational Biology Interdisciplinary Working Groups; Council on Epidemiology and Prevention. Contemporary definitions and classification of the cardiomyopathies: an American Heart Association Scientific Statement from the Council on Clinical Cardiology, Heart Failure and Transplantation Committee; Quality of Care and Outcomes Research and Functional Genomics and Translational Biology Interdisciplinary Working Groups; and Council on Epidemiology and Prevention. Circulation. 2006;113:1807-1816.

5. Elliott P, Andersson B, Arbustini E, Bilinska Z, Cecchi F, Charron P et al. Classification of the cardiomyopathies: a position statement from the European Society of Cardiology Working Group on

Myocardial and Pericardial Diseases. Eur Heart J. 2008; 29:270-276.

6. Thambo JB, Dos Santos P and Choussat A. Heart failure in infants and newborns. Encycl Méd Chir (Editions Scientifiques et Médicales Elsevier SAS, Paris, all rights reserved), Cardiology, 11-940- B-30, 2002, 15 p.

7. Sidi D and Bonnet D. Myocardial disease in children. Encycl Méd Chir (Editions Scientifiques et Médicales Elsevier SAS, Paris, all rights reserved), Pediatrics, 4-071-A-41, Cardiology, 11-022-A-10, 2000, 11 p.

8. Lipshultz SE, Sleeper LA, Towbin JA, Lowe AM, Orav EJ, Cox GF et al. The incidence of pediatric cardiomyopathy in two regions of the United States. N Engl J Med. 2003;348:1647- 1655.

9. Arola A, Jokinen E, Ruuskanen O, Saraste M, Pesonen E, Kuusela AL, et al. Epidemiology of idiopathic cardiomyopathies in children and adolescents: a nationwide study in Finland. Am J Epidemiol. 1997; 146:385-393.

10. Nugent AW, Daubeney PE, Chondros P, Carlin JB, Cheung M, Wilkinson LC et al. The epidemiology of childhood cardiomyopathy in Australia. National Australian Childhood Cardiomyopathy Study. N Angl Med. 2003 Apr 24; 348(17): 1639-46.

11. Oh JH, Hong YM, Choi JY, Kim SJ, Jung JW, Sohn SI et al. Idiopathic cardiomyopathies in Korean children. -9 Year Korean Multicenter Study. Circ J. 2011; 75(9):2228-34.

12. Daubeney PE , Nugent AW, Chondros P, Carlin JB, Colan SD, Cheung M et al. Clinical features and outcomes of childhood dilated cardiomyopathy: results from a national population-based study. Circulation. 2006 Dec 12; 114(24):2671-8.

13. Lamberti A, Fermont L, Batisse A. Idiopathic non-obstructive

cardiomyopathies in children. Ann Pédiat.1981; 18 :152-156.

14. Batisse A. Cardiologie Pédiatrique Pratique. 2002. p : 178-179.

15. Curtiss C, CohnJN, Vrobel T, Franciosa JA. Role of the reninangiotensin system in the systemic vasoconstriction of chronic congestive heart failure. Circulation 1978;58:763-770.

16. Dzau VJ. Local contractile and growth modulators in the myocardium. Clin Cardiol 1993; 16 (5 suppl 2): II5-II9.

17. Fifer MA, Molina CR, Quiroz AC, Giles TD, Herrmann HC, De Scheerder IR et al. Hemodynamic and renal effects of atrial natriuretic peptide in congestive heart failure. Am J Cardiol 1990; 65: 211-216.

18. Iacob D, Butnariu A, Leucuţa DC, Samaşca G, Deleanu D, Lupan I. Evaluation of NTproBNP in children with heart failure younger than 3 ye ars old. Rom J Intern Med. 2017 Jun 1;55(2):69-74.

19. Şahin M, Portakal O, Karagöz T, Hasçelik G, Özkutlu S. Diagnostic performance of bnp and nt-probnp measurements in children with heart failure based on congenital heart defects and cardiomyopathies. Clin biochem 2010; 43:1278-1281.

20. Harmon WG, Sleeper LA, Cuniberti L, Messere J, Colan SD, Orav EJ et al. Treating children with idiopathic dilated cardiomyopathy (From the Pediatric Cardiomyopathy Registry). Am J Cardiol. 2009; 104:281-6.

21. Lamberti. A, Ferment L, Batisse A. Idiopathic non-obstructive myocardiopathies in children. Ann Pedia 1981;285 :366-69.

22. Greenwood RO, Nadas AS, Fyler DC. The clinical course of primary myocardial disease in infants and children. Am Heart J 1976; 5: 549-60.

23. Pettersen MD. Cardiomyopathies commonly encountered in the teenage years and their presentation. Pedia Clin North Am. 2014;

61:173-86.

24. Han YY1, Zhai SB, Sun JH, Nie S, Yin FY. Clinical analysis of 68 cases of childhood dilated cardiomyopathy. Zhongguo Dang Dai Er Ke Za Zhi (2011 Feb), 13(2):135-7.

25. Lopez L, Colan SD, Frommelt PC, Ensing GJ, Kendall K, Younoszai AK, et al. Recommendations for quantification methods during the performance of a pediatric echocardiogram: a report from the Pediatric Measurements Writing Group of the American Society of Echocardiography Pediatric and Congenital Heart Disease Council. J Am SocEchocardiogr. (2010), 23:465-495.

26. Selamet Tierney ES, Hollenbeck-Pringle D, Lee CK, Altmann K, Dunbar-Masterson C, Golding F et al. Reproducibility of left ventricular dimension versus volume measurements in pediatric patients with dilated cardiomyopathy. Circ Cardiovasc Imaging. (2017 Nov),10(11).pii:e006007.

27. D'Oronzio U, Senn O, Biaggi P, Gruner C, Jenni R, Tanner FC, et al. Right heart assessment by echocardiography: gender and body size matters. J Am Soc Echocardiogr. (2012), 25:1251-1258.

28. Agha HM, Ibrahim H, El Satar IA, El Rahman NA, El Aziz DA, Salah Z et al. Forgotten Right Ventricle in Pediatric Dilated Cardiomyopathy. Pediatr Cardiol (2017 Apr), 38(4):819-827.

29. Zhang Y, He L, Cai J, Lv T, Yi Q, Xu Y. Measurements in Pediatric Patients with Cardiomyopathies: Comparison of Cardiac Magnetic Resonance Imaging and Echocardiography. Cardiology (2015), 131(4):245-50.

30. Liu G, Yang X, Su Y, Xu J, Wen Z. Cardiovascular magnetic resonance imaging findings in children with myocarditis. Chin Med J (Engl). (2014), 127(21):3700-5.

31. Raimondi F , Iserin F , Raisky O , Laux D , Bajolle F , Boudjemline Y. Myocardial inflammationon cardiovascularmagnetic resonance predicts left ventricular function recovery in children with recent dilated cardiomyopathy. Eur Heart J Cardiovasc Imaging (2015 Jul), 16(7):756-62.

32. Etesami M, Gilkeson RC, Rajiah P. Utility of late gadolinium enhancement in pediatric cardiac MRI. Pediatr Radiol.2016; 46:1096-113.

33. Daly KP, Marshall AC, Vincent JA, Zuckerman WA, Hoffman TM, Canter CE, et al. Endomyocardial biopsy and selective coronary angiography are low-risk procedures in pediatric heart transplant recipients: Results of a multicenter experience. J Heart Lung Transplant (2012), 31:398-409.

34. Leone O, Veinot JP, Angelini A, Baandrup UT, Basso C, Berry G et al . 2011 consensus statement on endomyocardial biopsy from the Association for European Cardiovascular Pathology and the Society for Cardiovascular Pathology. Cardiovasc Pathol (2012), 21:245-274.

35. Caforio AL, Pankuweit S, Arbustini E, Basso C, Gimeno-Blanes J, Felix SB, et al. European Society of Cardiology Working Group on Myocardial and Pericardial Diseases. Current state of knowledge on aetiology, diagnosis, management, and therapy of myocarditis: A position statement of the European Society of Cardiology Working Group on Myocardial and Pericardial Diseases. Eur Heart J (2013),34:2636-2648. 2648a-2648d.

36. Ghelani SJ, Spaeder MC, Pastor W, Spurney CF, Klugman D. Demographics, trends, and outcomes in pediatric acute myocarditis in the United States, 2006 to 2011. Circ Cardiovasc Qual Outcomes 2012; 5:622-627.

37. Gesuete V, Ragni L, Prandstraller D, Oppido G, Formigari R, Gargiulo GD et al. Dilated cardiomyopathy presenting in childhood: aetiology, diagnostic approach, and clinical course. Cardiology in the Young (2010), 20:680-685.

38. Brighenti M, Donti A, Gagliardi MG, Maschietto N, Marini D, Lombardi M et al. Endomyocardial Biopsy Safety and Clinical Yield in Pediatric Myocarditis: An Italian Perspective. Catheterization and Cardiovascular Interventions(2016), 87:762-767.

39. Nishikawa T, Uto K, Kanai S, Oda H, Kawamura S, Nakanishi T. Histopathological aspects of cardiac biopsy in pediatric patients with dilated cardiomyopathy. Pediatrics International (2011), 35: 350-353.

40. Zhorne D, Petit CJ, Ing FF, Justino H, Jefferies JL, Dreyer WJ et al. A 25-year experience of endomyocardial biopsy safety in infants. Catheter Cardiovasc Interv (2013), 82:797-801.

41. Bostan OM, Cil E. Dilated cardiomyopathy in childhood: prognostic features and outcome. Acta Cardiol (2006), 61: 169-174.

42. Kelly DP, Strauss AW. Inherited cardiomyopathies. NEngl J Med (1994), 330: 913-919.

43. Sidi D, Munnich A. Cardiopaediatrics and genetics: a collaboration that is beginning to bear fruit. Editorial. Arch Pédiatr (1994), 1: 458-462.

44. rochu JN, Piriou N, Toquet C, Bressollette C, Valleix F, Le Tourneau T, et al. Myocarditis. La Revue de médecine interne (2012), 33: 567-574.

45. De Bem RS, Da Ro Sa Utiyama SR, Nisihara RM, Fortunato JA, Tondo JA, Carmes ER et al. Celiac disease prevalence in brazilian dilated cardiomyopathy patients. Dig Dis Sci (2006), 51:1016-9.

46. Mahfoud F, Gärtner B, Kindermann M, Ukena C, Gadomski K,

Klingel K, et al. Virus serology in patients with suspected myocarditis: utility or futility. Eur Heart J (2011), 32:897-903.

47. Blauwet LA, Cooper LT. Myocarditis. Prog Cardiovasc Dis 2010; 52:274-88.

48. Amat di Sanfilipo C, Taylor MRG, Mestroni L, Botto LD, Longo N. Cardiomyopathy and carnitine deficiency. Mol Gen Metab 2008; 94: 162- 6.

49. Shaw T, Elliiott P, Mckenna WJ. Dilated cardiomyopathy genetically heterogeneous disease. Lancet 2002; 360: 654-5.

50. Richard P, Fressart V, Charron P, Hainque B. Genetics of hereditary cardiomyopathies. Pathologie Biologie 58 (2010) 343-352.

51. Tesson F, Charron P, Schwartz K, Komajda M. Génétique des cardiomyopathies dilatées. médecine/sciences. 1999 ; 15 : 369-75.

52. Olson TM, Michels VV, Thibodeau SN, Tai YS, Keating MT. Actin mutations in dilated cardiomyopathy, a heritable form of heart failure. Science 1998; 280: 750-2.

53. Bowles KR, Gajarski R, Porter P, Goytia V, Bachinski L, Roberts R, et al. Gene mapping of familial autosomal dominant dilated cardiomyopathy to chromosome 10q21-23. J Clin Invest 1996; 98: 1355-60.

54. Li D, Tapscoft T, Gonzalez O, Burch P, Quin˜ones M, Zoghbi W et al. Desmin mutation responsible for idiopathic dilated cardiomyopathy. Circulation 1999;100(5):461-4.

55. Villard E, Duboscq-Bidot L, Charron P, Benaiche A, Conraads V, Sylvius N, et al. Mutation screening in dilated cardiomyopathy: prominent role of the beta myosin heavy chain gene. Eur Heart J 2005;26(8):794-803.

56. Watkins H. Genetic clues to disease pathways in hypertrophic and

dilated cardiomyopathies. Circulation 2003; 107(10):1344-6.

57. Zhang Y, Wang Y, Zhai M, Gan T, Zhao X, Zhang R et al. Influence of LGALS3 gene polymorphisms on susceptibility and prognosis of dilated cardiomyopathy in a Northern Han Chinese population. Gene. 2018 Feb 5;642:293-298.

58. Masarone D, Valente F, Rubino M, Vastarella R , Gravino R, Rea A et al. Pediatric Heart Failure: A Practical Guide to Diagnosis and Management. Pediatr Neonatol. 2017 Aug;58(4):303-312.

M. Jayaprasad N. Heart failure in children. Heart Views 2016;17:92-9.Kirk R, Dipchand AI, Rosenthal DN, Addonizio L, Burch M, Chrisant The international Society for Heart and Lung Transplantation Guidelines for the management of pediatric heart failure: executive summary. J Heart Lung Transplant. 2014 Sep;33(9):888-909.

59. Hussey AD, Weintraub RG. Drug treatment of heart failure in children: focus on recent recommendations from the ISHLT Guidelines for the Management of Pediatric Heart Failure. Paediatr Drugs 2016;18:89e99.

60. Alabed S, Sabouni A, Al Dakhoul S, Bdaiwi Y, Frobel-Mercier AK. Beta- blockers for congestive heart failure in children. Cochrane Database Syst Rev 2016;(1):CD007037.

61. Hoffman TM, Wernovsky G, Atz AM, Kulik TJ, Nelson DP, Chang AC, et al. Efficacy and safety of milrinone in preventing low cardiac output syndrome in infants and children after corrective surgery for congenital heart disease. Circulation 2003;107: 996-1002.

62. Egan JR, Clarke AJ, Williams S, Cole AD, Ayer J, Jacobe S, et al. Levosimendan for low cardiac output: A pediatric experience. J Intensive Care Med 2006;21:183-7.

63. Rognoni A, Lupi A, Lazzero M, Bongo AS, Rognoni G. Levosimendan: from basic science to clinical trials. Recent Pat Cardiovasc Drug Discov 2011;6:9e15.

64. Ratnapalan S, Griffiths K, Costei AM, Benson L, Koren G. Digoxin- carvedilol interactions in children. J Pediatr 2003;142:572-4.

65. Mets G, Panzer J, De Wolf D, Bové T. An Alternative Strategy for Bridge-to-Transplant/Recovery in Small Children with Dilated Cardiomyopathy. Pediatr Cardiol (2017) 38:902-908.

66. Cooper DS, Jacobs JP, Moore L, Stock A, Gaynor JW, Chancy T et al Cardiac extracorporeal life support: state of the art in 2007. Cardiol Young (2007) 17 (Suppl 2):104-115.

67. Gournay V, Hauet Q (2014) Mechanical circulatory support for infants and small children. Arch Cardiovasc Dis 107(6-7):398-405.

68. Almond CS, Singh TP, Gauvreau K, Piercey GE, Fynn-Thompson F, Rycus PT et al. Extracorporeal membrane oxygenation for bridge to heart transplantation among children in the United States: analysis of data from the organ procurement and transplant network and extracorporeal life support organization registry. Circulation (2011) 123(25):2975-2984.

69. Merrill ED, Schoeneberg L, Sandesara P, Molitor-Kirsch E, O'Brien J Jr, Dai H et al. Outcomes after prolonged extracorporeal membrane oxygenation support in children with cardiac disease-extracorporeal life support organization registry study. J Thorac Cardiovasc Surg (2014) 148(2):582-588.

70. Almond CS, Morales DL, Blackstone EH, Turrentine MW, Imamura M, Massicotte MP et al. Berlin Heart EXCOR pediatric ventricular assist device for bridge to heart transplantation in US children. Circulation (2013) 127(16):1702-1711.

M. Zafar F, Castleberry C, Khan MS, Mehta V, Bryant R 3rd, Lorts A et al. Pediatric heart transplant waiting list mortality in the era of ventricular assist devices. J Heart Lung Transplant (2015) 34(1):82-88. Brancaccio G, Amodeo A, Ricci Z, Morelli S, Gagliardi MG, Iacobelli R et al. Mechanical assist device as a bridge to heart transplantation in children less than 10 kilograms. Ann Thorac Surg(2010) 90(1):58-62 Karimova A, Van Doorn C, Brown K, Giardini A, Kostolny M, Mathias M et al. Mechanical bridging to orthotopic heart transplantation in children weighing less than 10 kg: feasibility and limitations. Eur J Cardio-Thorac Surg (2011) 39(3):304-309. Schranz D, Rupp S, Muller M, Schmidt D, Bauer A, Valeske K et al. Pulmonary artery banding in infants and young children with left ventricular dilated cardiomyopathy: a novel therapeutic strategy before heart transplantation. J Heart Lung Transplant (2013) 32(5):475-481. Pincott ES, Ridout D, Brocklesby M, McEwan A, Muthurangu V, Burch A randomized study of autologous bone marrow- derived stem cells in pediatric cardiomyopathy. J Heart Lung Transplant. 2017 Aug; 36(8):837-844.

71. Moriguchi T, Koizumi K, Matsuda K, Harii N, -Goto J, Harada D et al. Plasma exchange for the patients with dilated cardiomyopathy in children is safe and effective in improving both cardiac function and daily activities. J Artif Organs (2017) 20:236-243.

72. Lewis AB, Chabot M. Outcome of infants and children with dilated cardiomyopathy. Am J Cardiol. 1991;68:365-369.

73. Tsirka AE, Trinkaus K, Chen SC, Lipshultz SE, Towbin JA, Colan SD, et al. Improved outcomes of pediatric dilated cardiomyopathy with utilization of heart transplantation. J Am Coll Cardiol. 2004;44:391-397.

74. Alexander PM1, Daubeney PE, Nugent AW, Lee KJ, Turner C, Colan SD et al. Long-Term Outcomes of Dilated Cardiomyopathy Diagnosed During Childhood Results From a National Population-Based Study of Childhood Cardiomyopathy. Circulation. 2013 Oct 29;128(18):2039-46

SUMMARY

CMD is the most common cardiomyopathy in children. Its incidence is difficult to estimate and requires the creation of national registries. Epidemiological data show that it is more common in infants, males and blacks. Looking for parental consanguinity or an affected family member is an important part of the history. Clinically, it generally presents as acute heart failure. Cardiac ultrasound confirms the diagnosis by showing a dilated heart that contracts poorly. Cardiac MRI is a powerful tool that not only confirms the diagnosis but also guides the search for the cause and predicts the prognosis. The main purpose of endomyocardial biopsy is to confirm viral myocarditis. CMD in children is classified into primary and secondary CMD. Primary DCMs are hereditary or metabolic in origin, whereas secondary DCMs may result from a left-sided obstruction, a long-standing left-to-right shunt, a rhythm or conduction disorder, a birth defect of the coronary arteries, or viral or autoimmune myocarditis. Treatment is based primarily on treating cardiac decompensation. Treatment of the cause is essential in cases of secondary DCM. In the case of primary DCM and in the absence of recovery, heart transplantation is the only hope of life.

TABLE OF CONTENTS

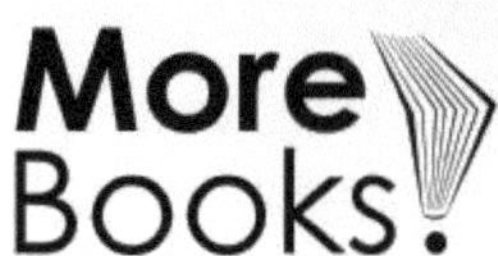

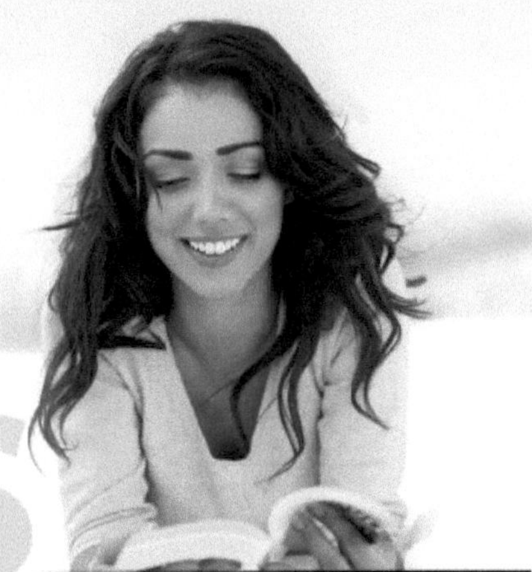

Buy your books fast and straightforward online - at one of world's fastest growing online book stores! Environmentally sound due to Print-on-Demand technologies.

Buy your books online at
www.morebooks.shop

Kaufen Sie Ihre Bücher schnell und unkompliziert online – auf einer der am schnellsten wachsenden Buchhandelsplattformen weltweit! Dank Print-On-Demand umwelt- und ressourcenschonend produziert.

Bücher schneller online kaufen
www.morebooks.shop

info@omniscriptum.com
www.omniscriptum.com

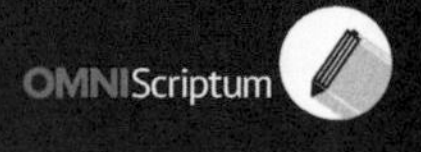

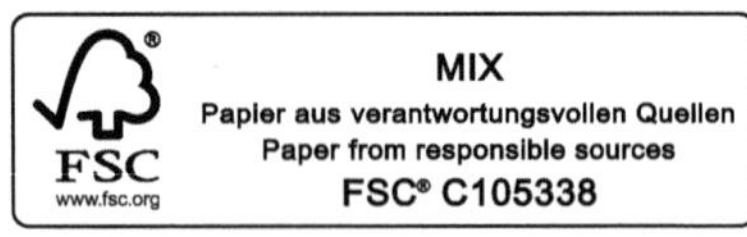

Printed by Books on Demand GmbH, Norderstedt / Germany